On the Way to Uncle George

A road-user education book
for parents and young children

Written by Jean Roberts

Illustrated by Colin Hale

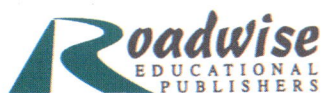

Roadwise
EDUCATIONAL PUBLISHERS

First published in Great Britain in 1995 by

Roadwise Educational Publishers
P O Box 4555
Halesowen West Midlands B63 4SY

Text Copyright © Jean Roberts 1995
Illustrations Copyright © Jean Roberts 1995
The Road Crossing Song © Jean Roberts 1995

British Cataloguing in Publication Data
A catalogue record for this book is available from the British Library

Printed in Great Britain by BPC Paulton Books Ltd Bristol

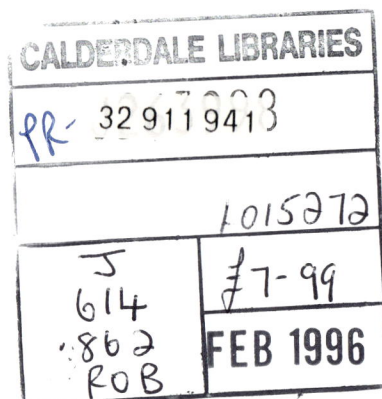

ISBN 0 9524272 0 6

ON THE WAY TO UNCLE GEORGE

Introductions

a Story

Questions

and
a Song to sing

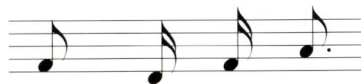

An audio cassette and the "On the Way" Music Activity Book for Teachers are available.

The series of "On the Way" books are available from all good bookshops. In case of difficulty please contact the publishers direct.

Roadwise Educational Publishers PO Box 4555 Halesowen West Midlands B63 4SY

INTRODUCTION TO "ON THE WAY" BOOKS

Road accidents happen every day. On average over 30 children a day and 200 children a week aged 6 and under are injured on the roads in the United Kingdom; almost half are pedestrians.

How can accidents to children be prevented?

Children need to learn to make safe choices. If children are to learn how to cross a road safely for themselves they need to be involved in the decision making process from an early age: all too often children are passive participants in the road crossing process - decisions being made by adults with children just 'walked' across the road.

This series of four books illustrates different types of road crossings and how to use them. Safe crossing procedures are demonstrated in each story showing how children can be involved in decisions of where and when it is safe to cross the road. When out walking with a child and having to cross a road the same teaching guidelines as in the stories can be applied; and remember, when crossing a road always hold the hand of the child so that decisions can be checked before action is taken.

Each book includes questions within the story and questions with pictures at the end which will help to assess the young child's understanding. These may not necessarily be used the first time the book is read, but when thought appropriate.

There is also a song to accompany the series, a verse and chorus are included in each book. You will have the complete song when you have all four books. An audio cassette and the "On the Way" Music Activity Book for Teachers are available.

A small investment of buying and using all four books could save your child's life.

James and his mother were out walking when suddenly a helicopter appeared and began to follow them......

This book has an interesting story designed to encourage adults and children to talk about subways and footbridges, emphasising that they are safe places to cross a road. On some pages there are *Roadwise Questions* These again can promote discussion.

At the end of the story there are pictures and questions which help the child to become aware of, and look for, footbridges and subways. One verse of the song is included at the end of the book and it is about crossing a road using a footbridge and subway.

Footbridges and subways are normally very safe places to use when crossing a road but, for a variety of reasons, adults sometimes try to cross busy roads rather than use a footbridge or subway. This is not good teaching and it is not safe practice. A child will often copy what an adult does and if a footbridge or subway is always used where available (even if it means walking a little farther) a child will probably come to recognise the importance of using safe places to cross the road. It may be helpful if the effort of using a footbridge or subway can be made to seem worthwhile, for example, what can be seen from the top of the bridge, birds flying, people working, a helicopter or plane?

The time taken for a child to recognise and look for subways and footbridges will vary, and children need to be questioned frequently about their responses to make sure that the child really is able to make safe decisions.

Footnote: Whilst acknowledging that subways may not always be safe places, it is generally much safer to use subways rather than attempt to cross a busy road.

ON THE WAY TO UNCLE GEORGE

"Ahhh..." shrieked James as he raced down the path on his bicycle. He was so busy rushing up and down the path that he didn't hear his mother calling him.

"James! James, lunch is ready!"

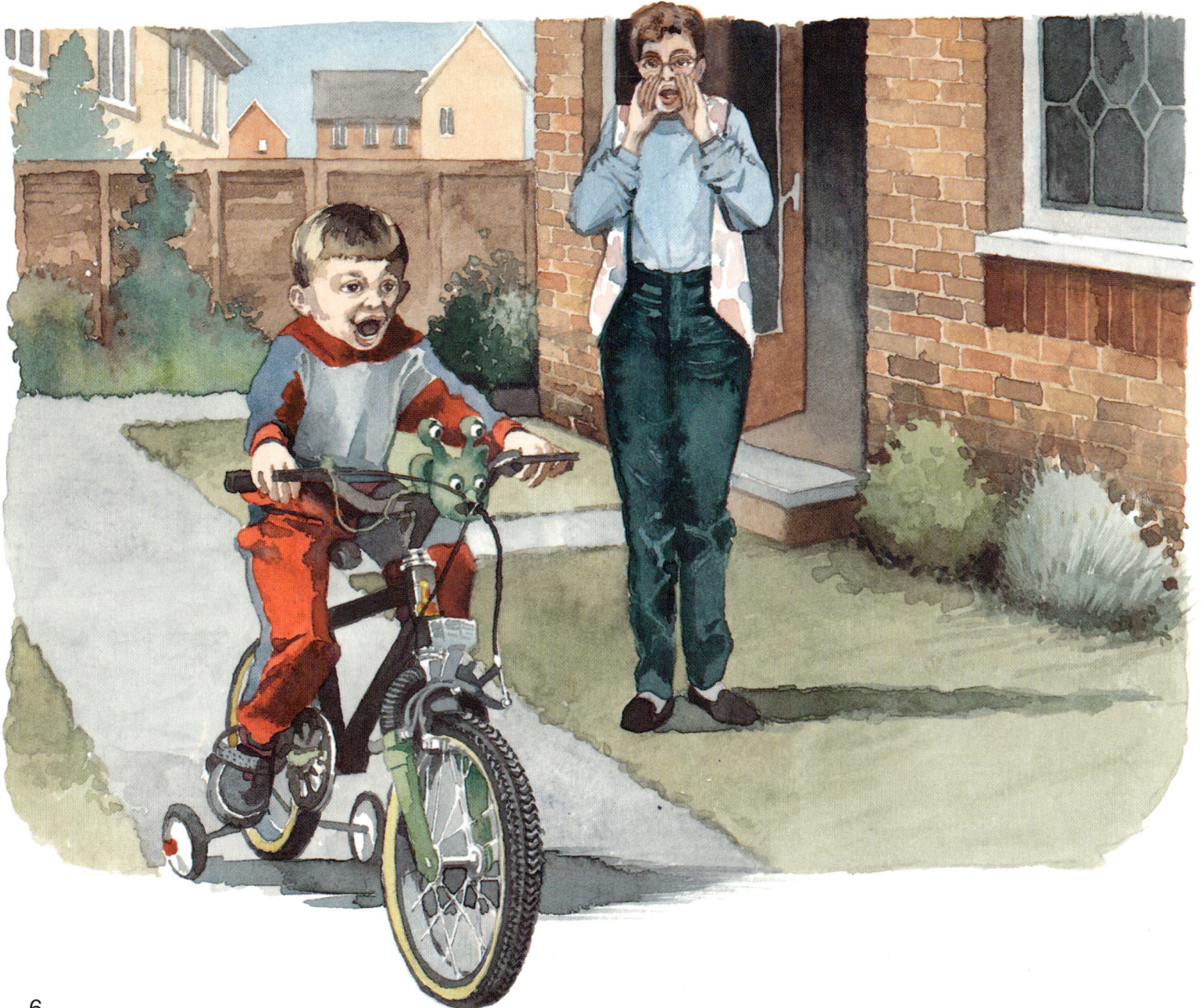

"It is such a lovely day that I thought we would visit Uncle George this afternoon," said mother. "What will you take to show Uncle George?"

James sat thinking.

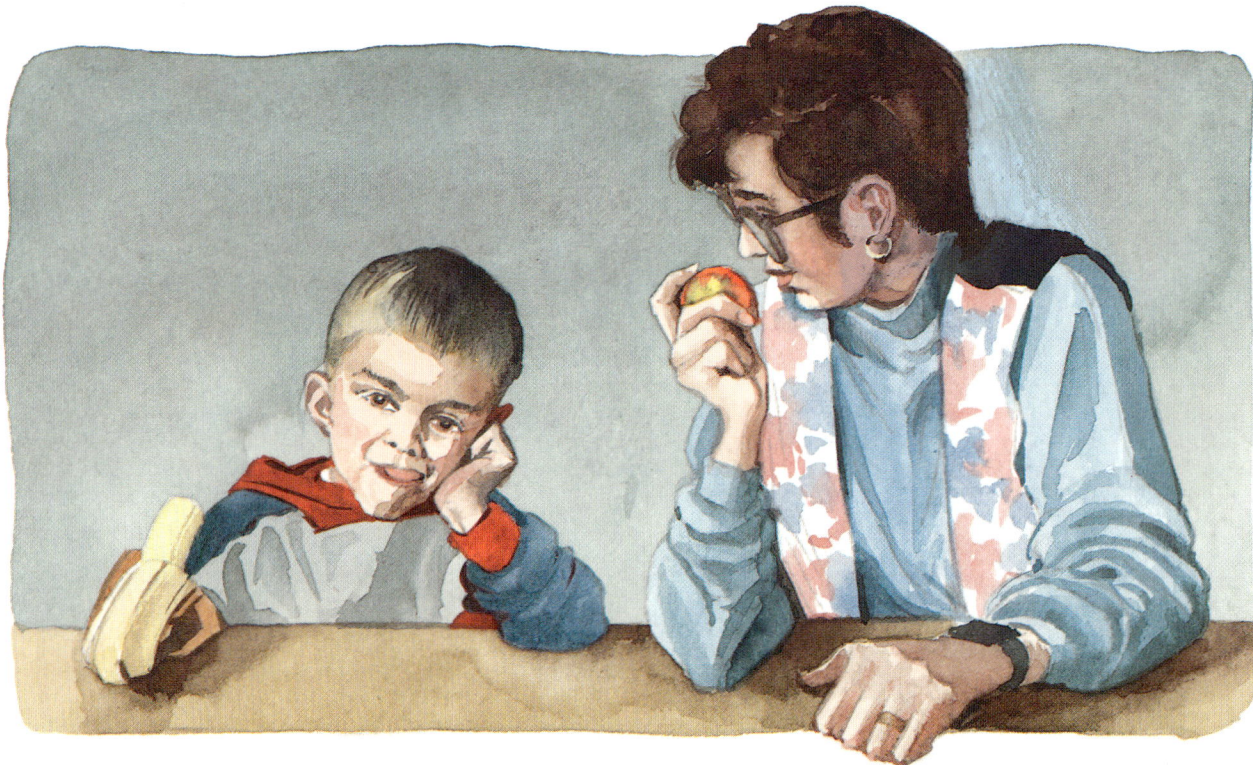

His eyes suddenly lit up. "I know," he said "we'll take the peacock feather we found the other day in the park. It has such lovely colours I'm sure he'd like to see it."

"That's a good idea," said mother, "we can also take him some of the little cakes we baked yesterday."

Uncle George lived near the city centre so they had to catch a train. They walked up to the station and waited for the train to arrive. "Here it is," said James.

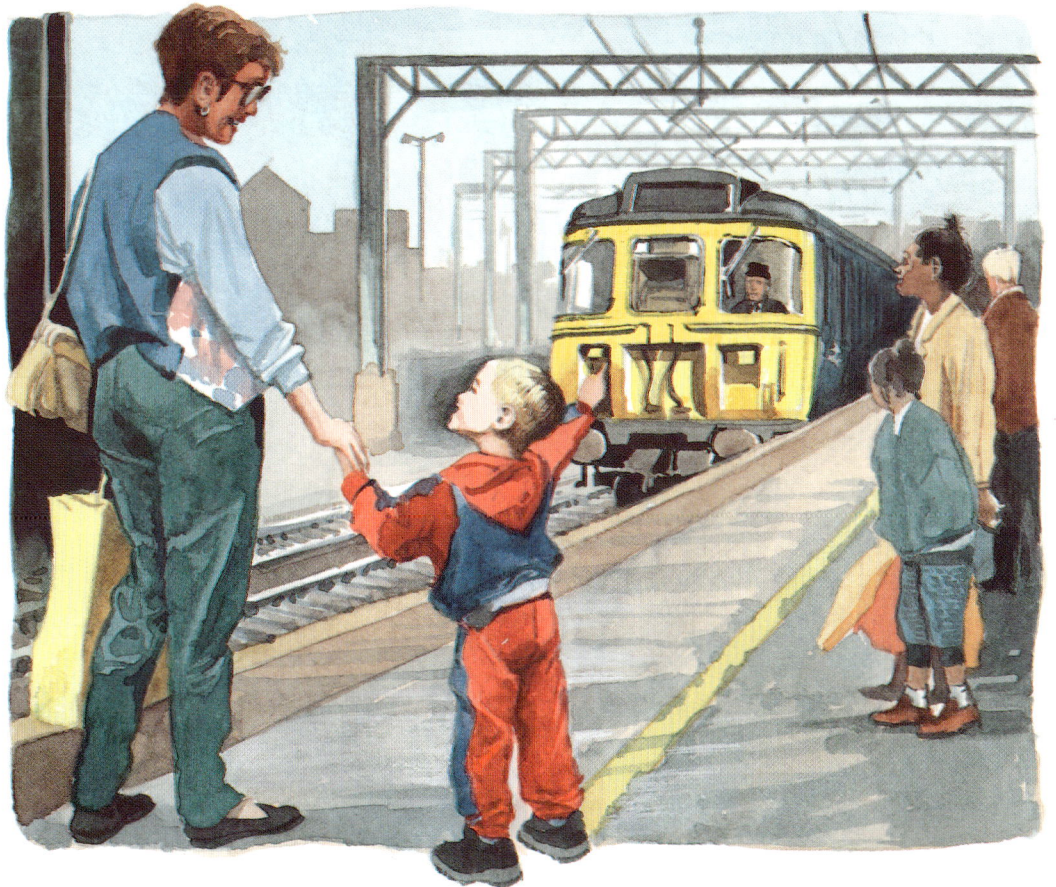

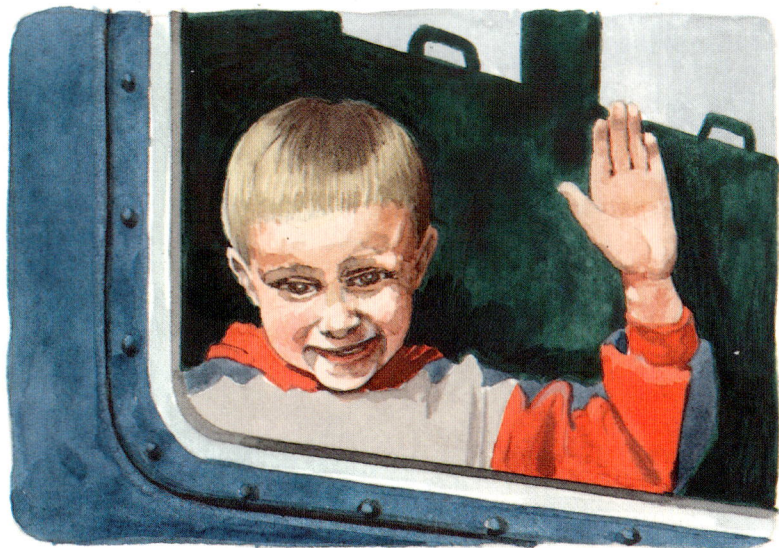

They got into the train, doors closed, the guard blew the whistle and they were on their way!

On leaving the station they had to cross a very busy main road, so James and his mother always used the footbridge. The footbridge took them high above the cars and lorries and brought them safely down on the other side of the road. James was feeling full of energy so they chose to walk up the steps.

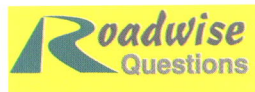

Roadwise Questions

Have you walked up a footbridge?

Did you walk up the steps?

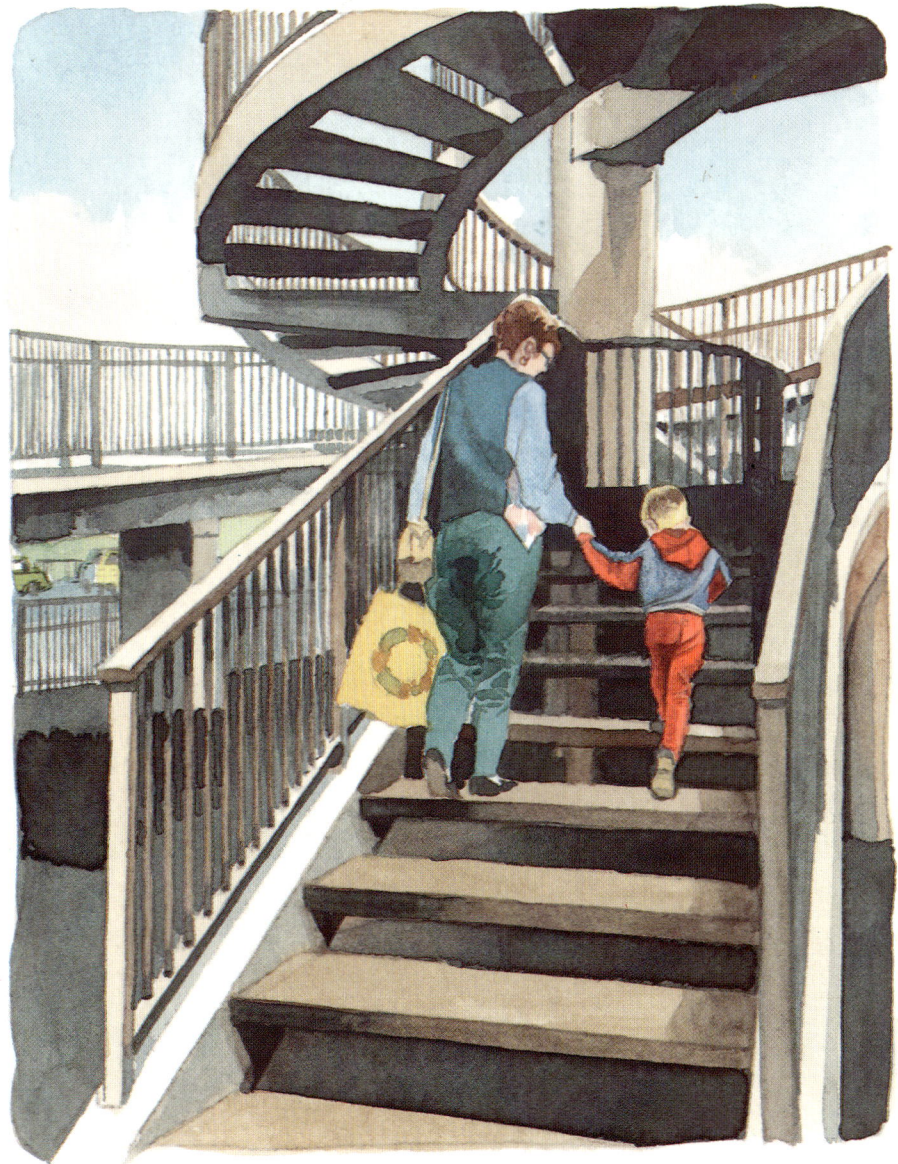

9

When they reached the top of the bridge they could see cars and lorries rushing past along the road below.

"Just as well we came this way," said James, "I don't think we'd ever have got across the road otherwise."

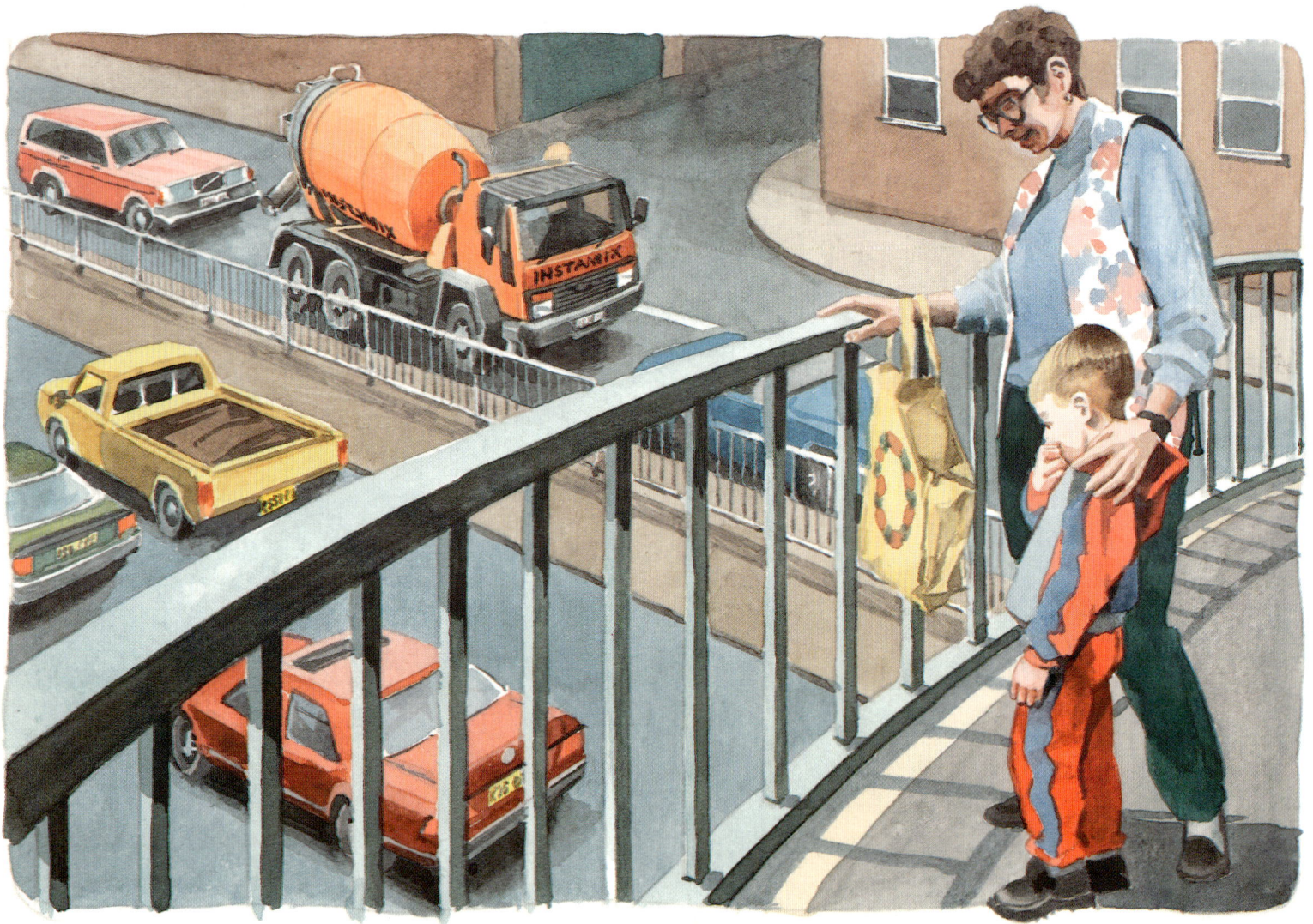

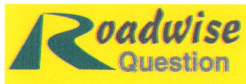

Roadwise Question When you were on a bridge did you see lots of cars and lorries rushing along the road?

10

"Wow! Look at that over there!" said James.

"Ooh!" said his mother, "it's a large crane and it's moving something towards us. Oh I can see it now, there are lots of long metal pipes." They watched the crane for several minutes before mother said that they must go on their way to see Uncle George.

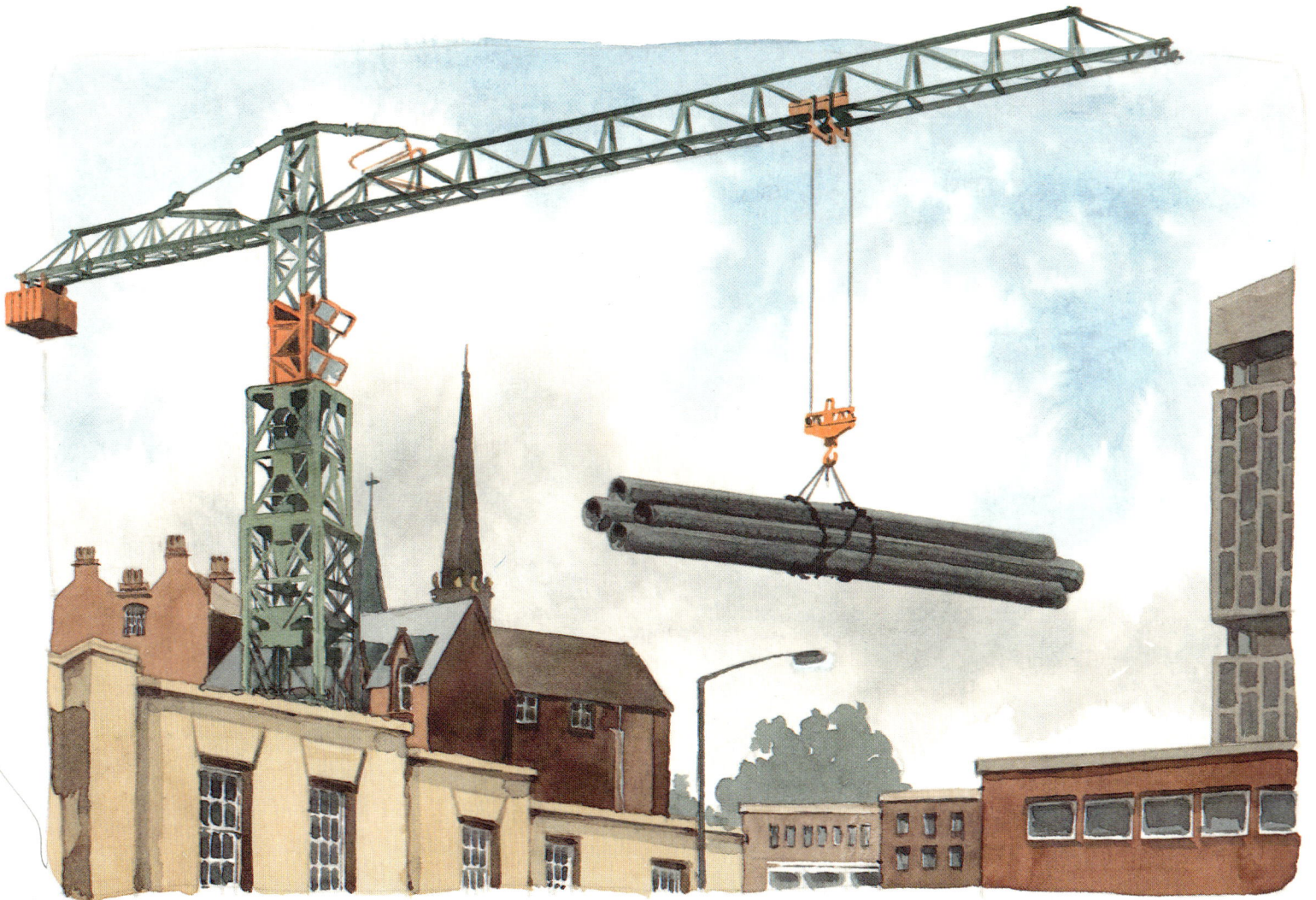

Roadwise Question What have you seen from the top of a footbridge?

Before they had taken more than a few steps James said, "Wait, I can hear something." He looked around. "There it is! It's a helicopter and it's coming towards us."

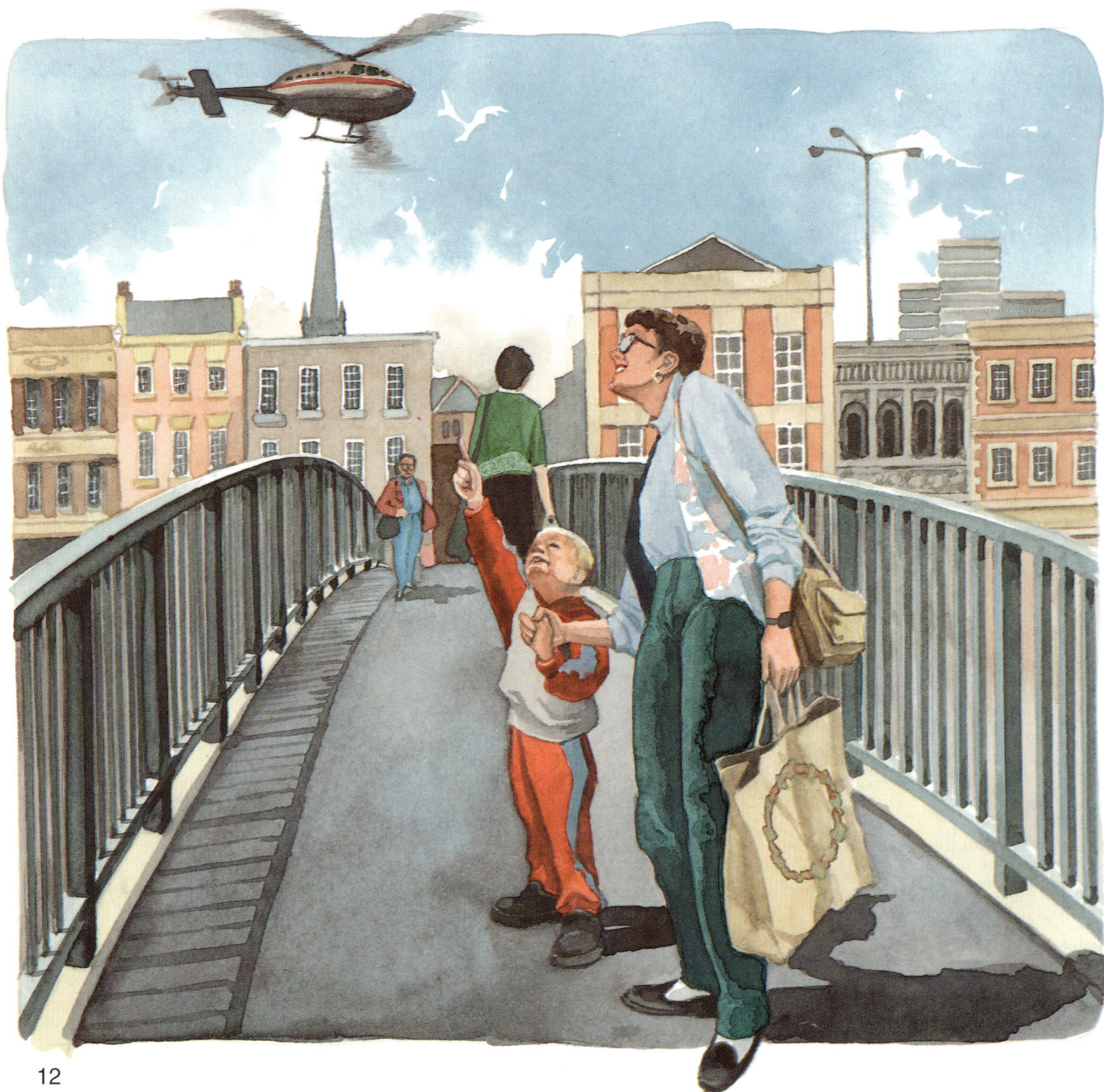

James wanted to stay and watch the helicopter, his mother kept pulling him so he had no choice but to walk with her.

"It's following us," said James. "Look, it's coming our way, I think it's going to show us the way to Uncle George's house."

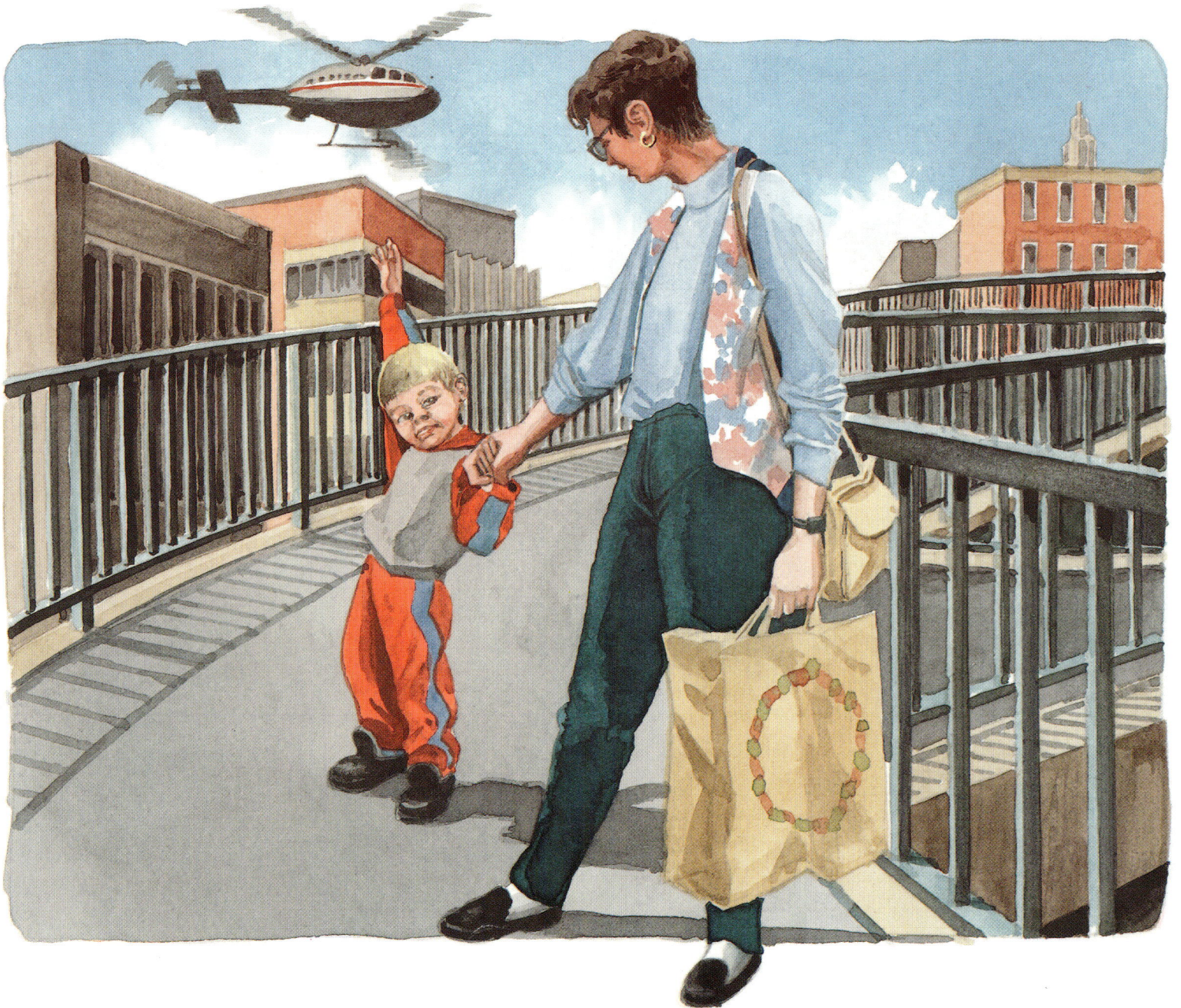

"We will use the subway and then we shall be near Uncle George's," said his mother.

The subway went underneath the road and, like the footbridge, it was a safe way to get to the other side of the road.

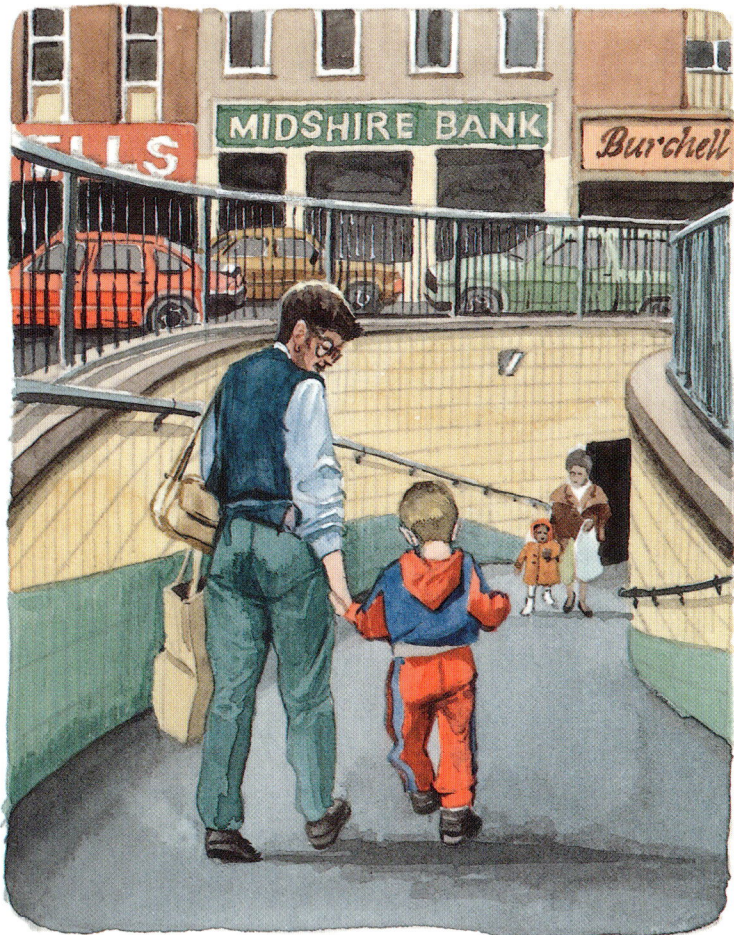

James wasn't keen to go down the steps so they chose to go down the slope into the subway. Cars, buses and lorries rumbled overhead.

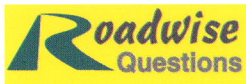

Roadwise Questions Have you walked through a subway?
Did you walk down the steps or the slope?

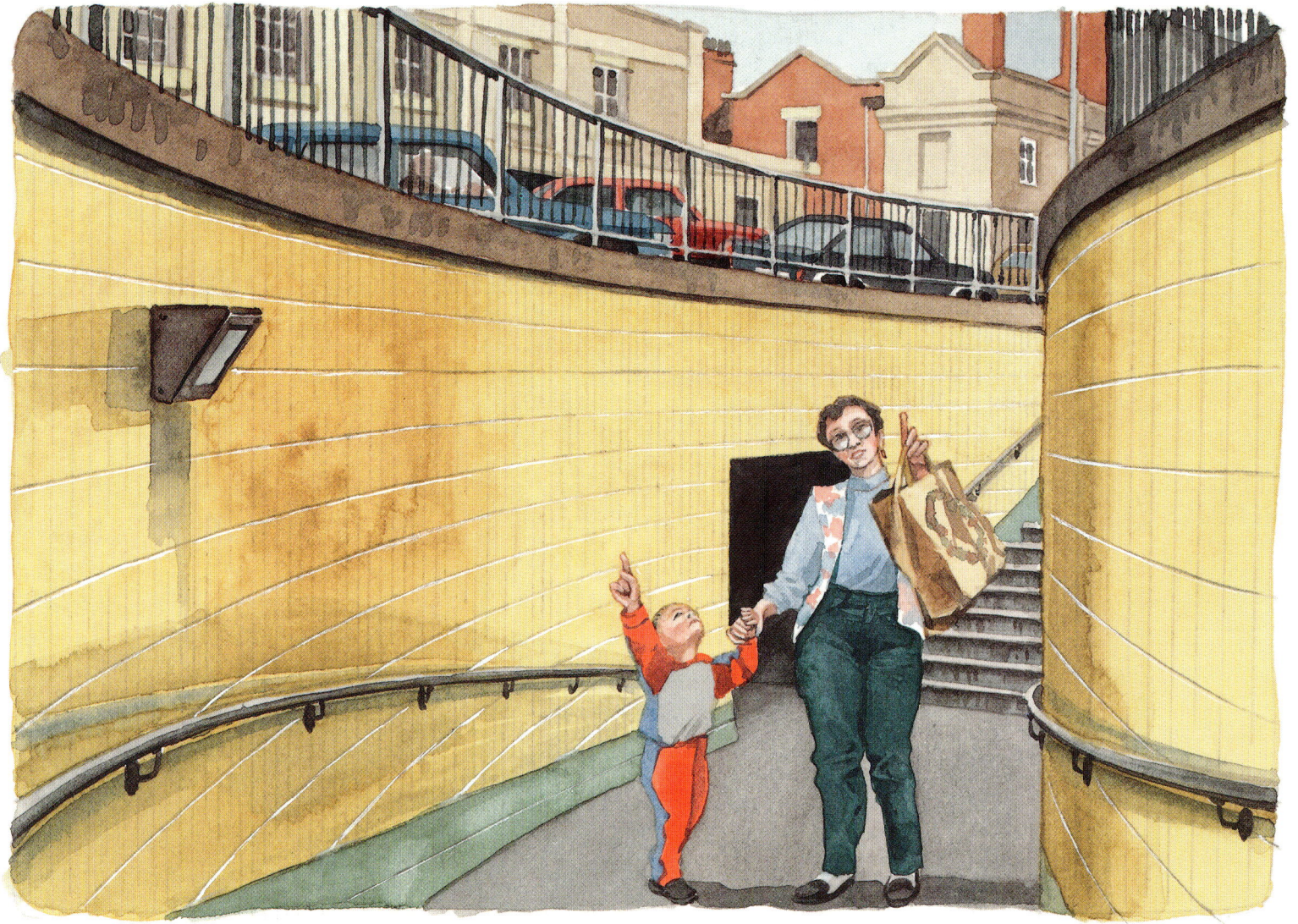

As they came up the other side of the subway James shouted, "There it is, it has followed us and I think it will show us the way to Uncle George's house."

"The helicopter does seem to have followed us," agreed his mother. "Look, now I can see the house where Uncle George lives."

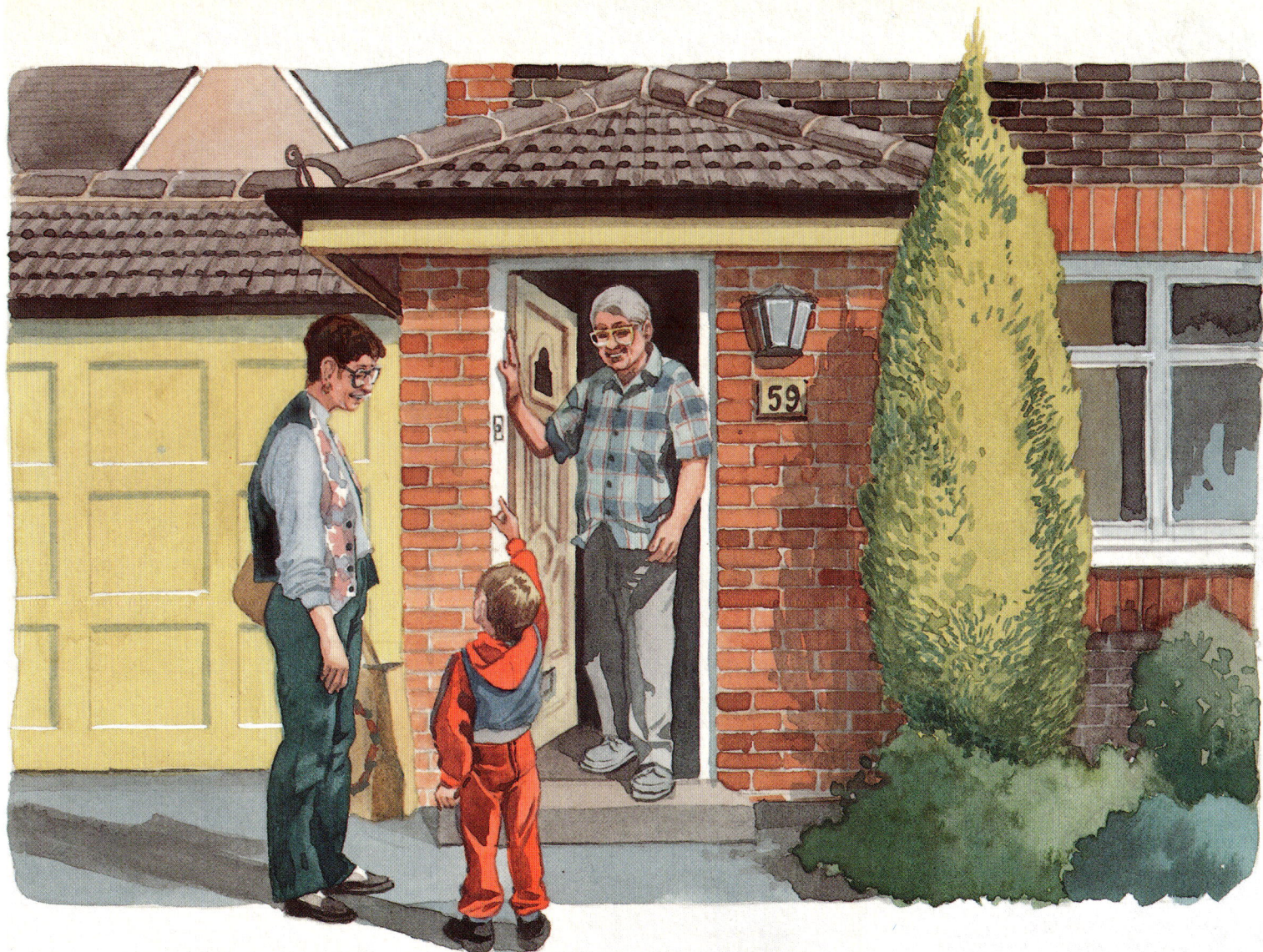

When they arrived at Uncle George's, Mother rang the bell and waited. Uncle George opened the door. "How lovely to see you! Come inside."

"Uncle George," said James pointing up to the sky excitedly, "you see this helicopter, well, it followed us all the way to your house! It even waited for us while we went down through the subway, and was there when we came up again."

"Well I never!" said Uncle George, surprised. "Oh look, it's moving off into the distance."

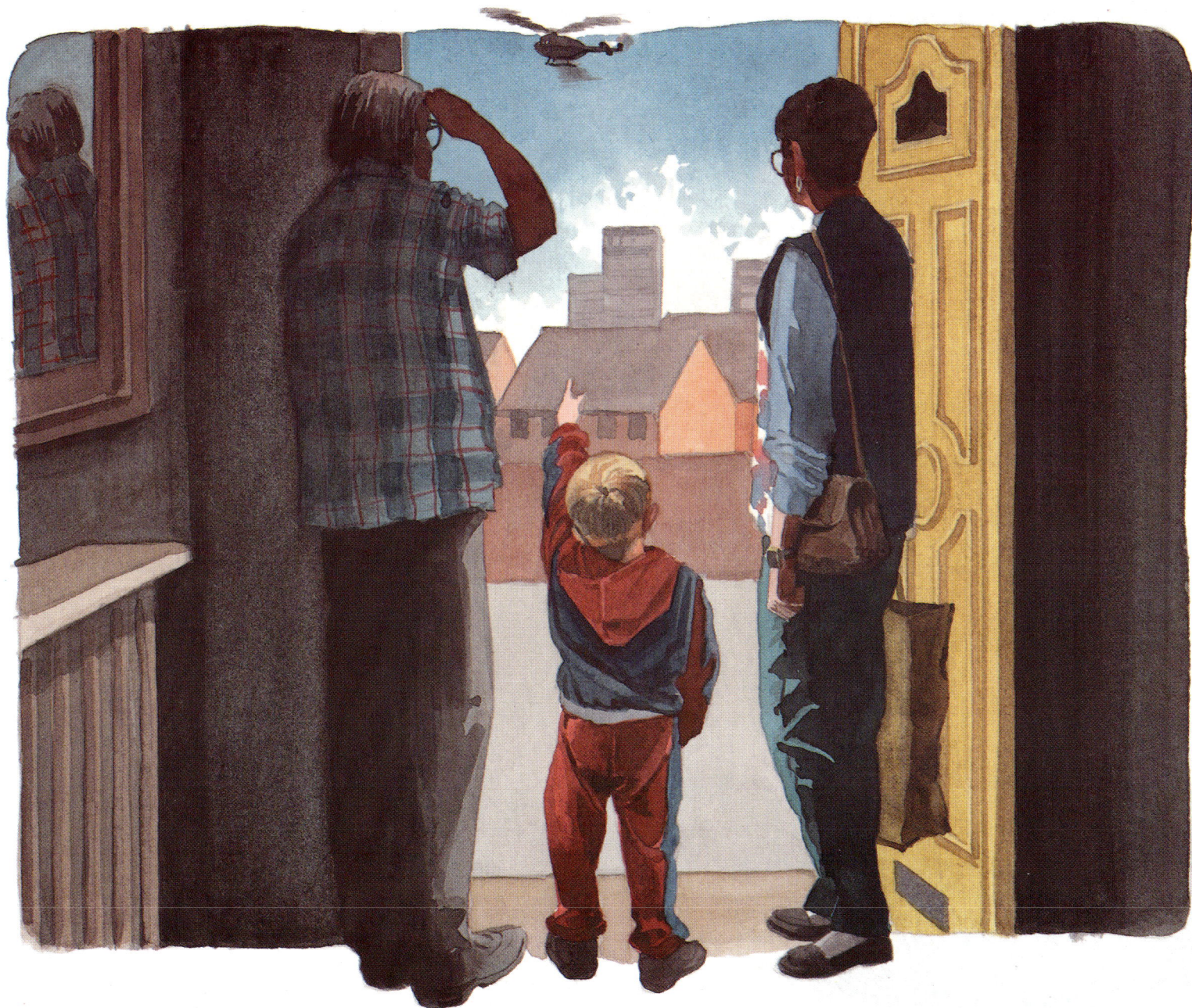

"Just what I told you," said James "it only came to show us the way to your house!"

James told Uncle George that they had seen a large crane moving long metal pipes.

"You must have seen that from the footbridge," said Uncle George. "You get a good view from up there and it is much safer than trying to cross such a busy road."

"Yes, there were lots of cars and lorries rushing past below, but we were safe on the bridge," said James.

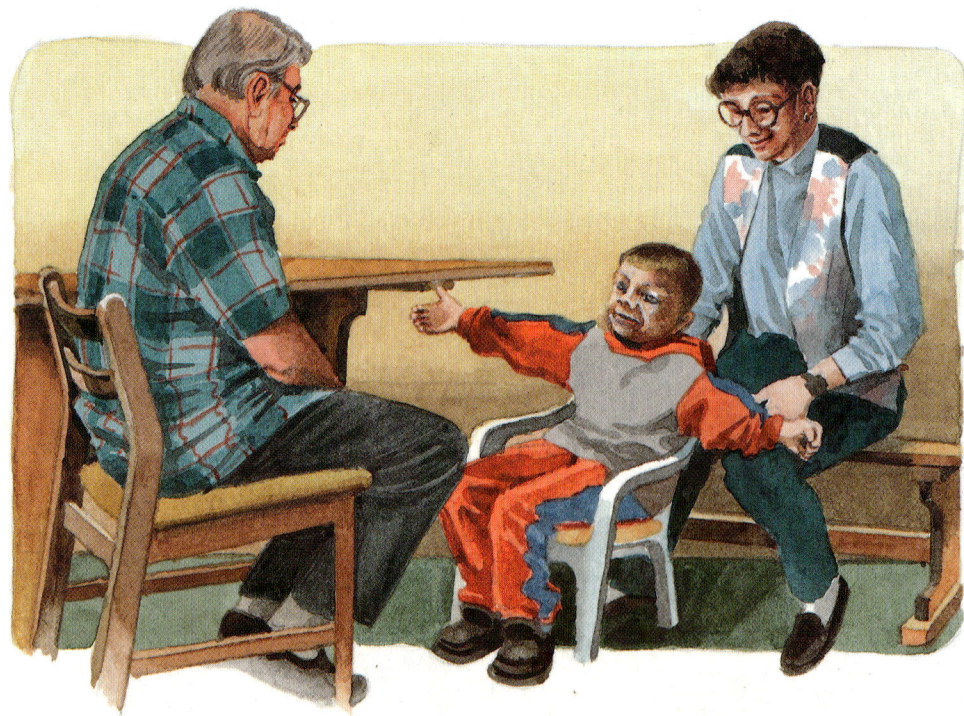

Uncle George got up to make a cup of tea for James's mother and himself and brought in some orange juice for James. He asked James if he had brought him anything to look at.

"I nearly forgot," said James as he dived into his mother's large bag. "Here is a peacock feather we found. Isn't it pretty?"

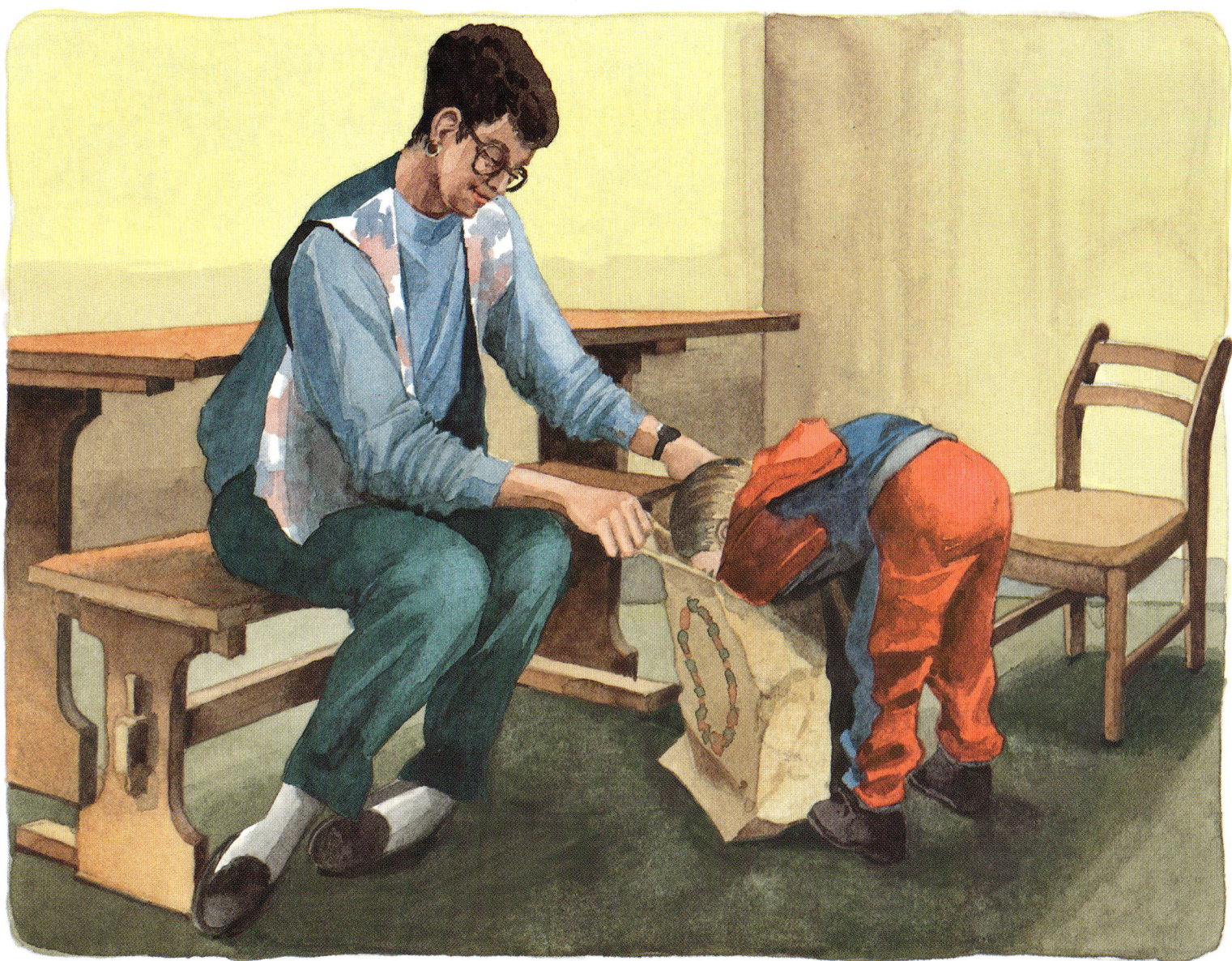

Uncle George admired the feather and then asked James if he had seen a real peacock.

"Only in pictures," said James "I'd like to see one showing off all his pretty coloured feathers."

"Well, one day we could all go to the country park: there are peacocks, hens, ponies, donkeys, pigs and lots more animals," said Uncle George.

"Ooh.. yes please," said James "I'd like that."

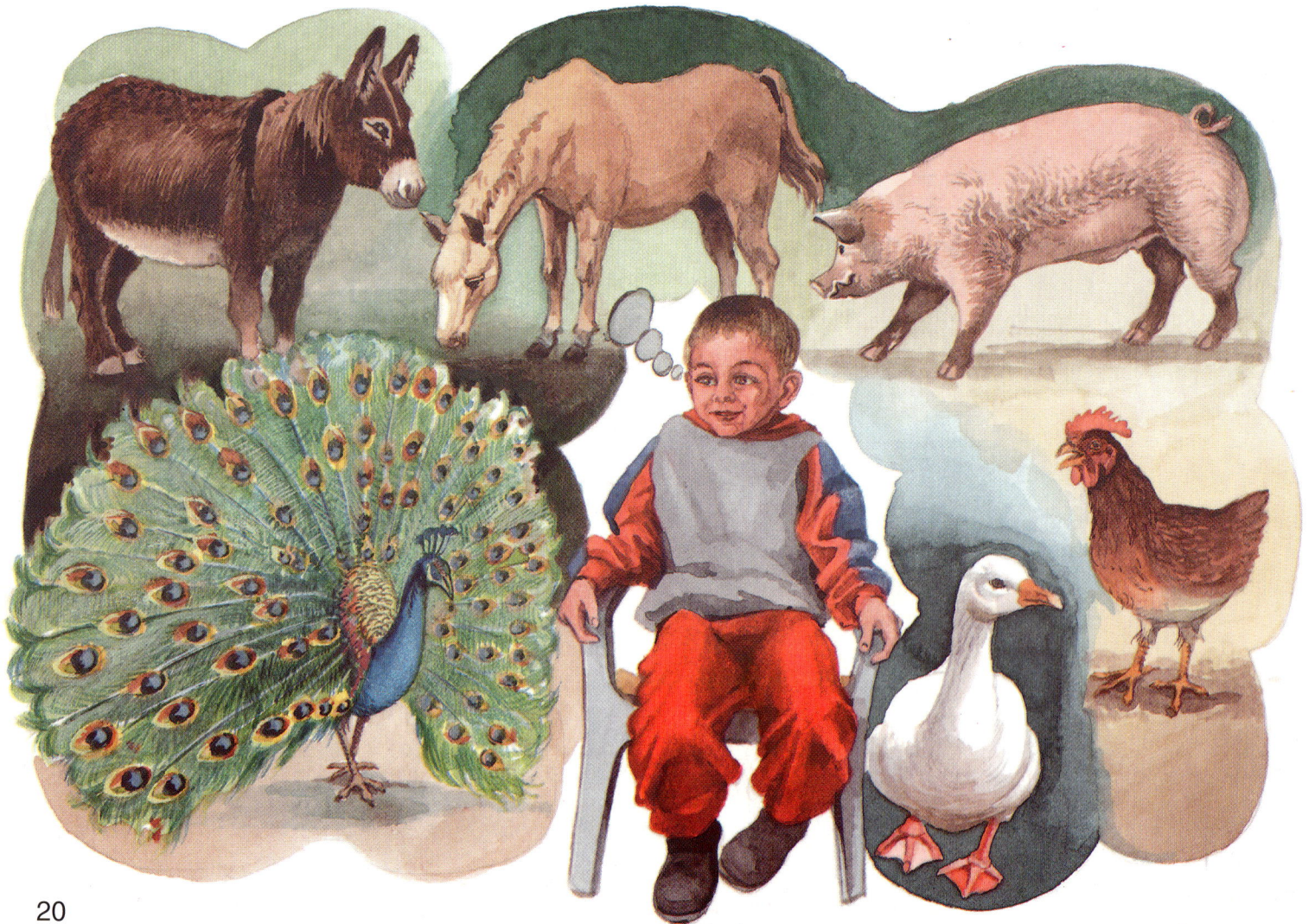

"Oh here are some cakes that Mother and I made yesterday," said James.

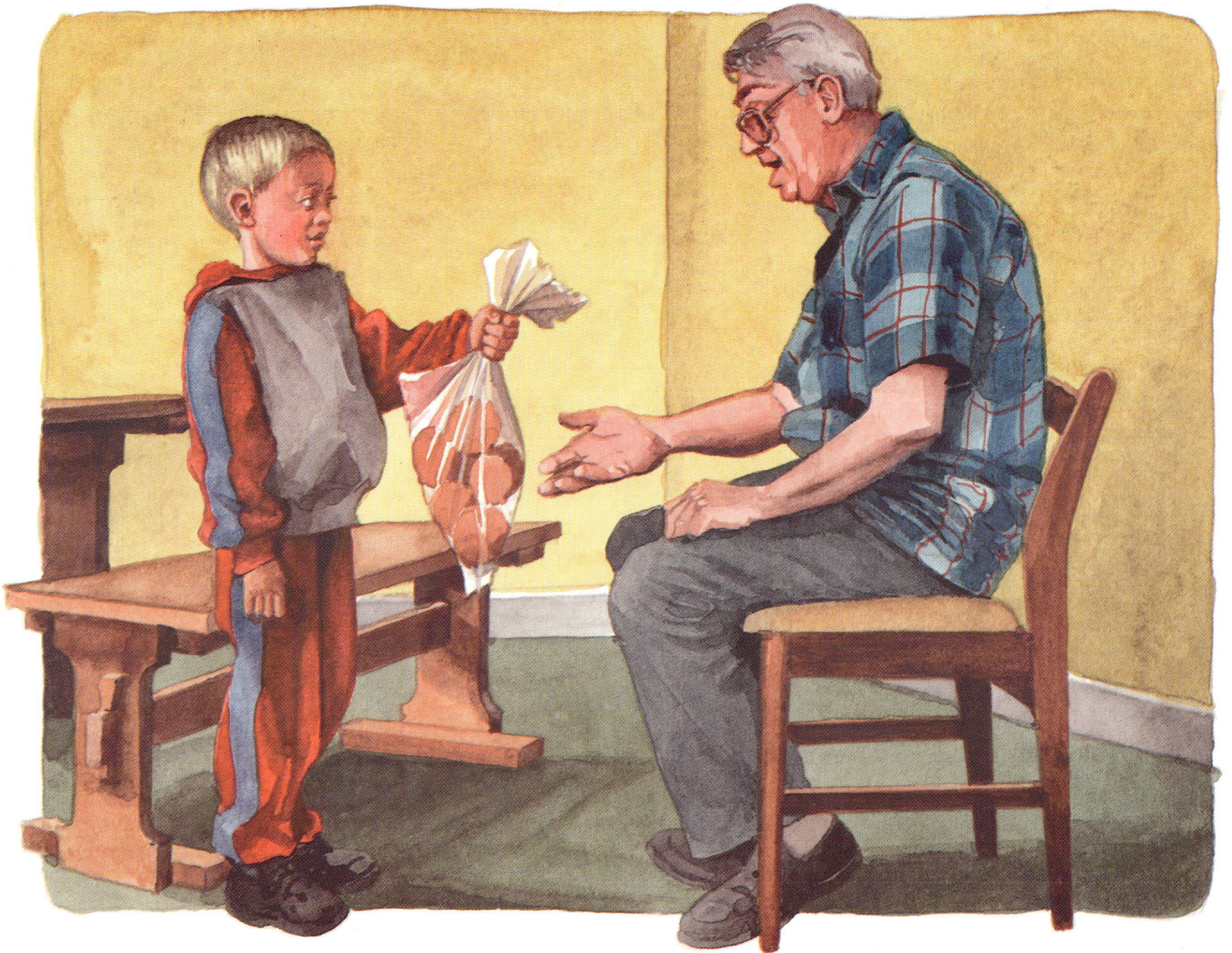

"Thank you very much," said Uncle George, "I will look forward to eating them, especially as you helped to make them, James."

"I think that we had better return home soon," said James's mother reluctantly.   They always enjoyed visiting Uncle George. Uncle George was not related to James but he was a friendly old gentleman whom they had got to know and love.

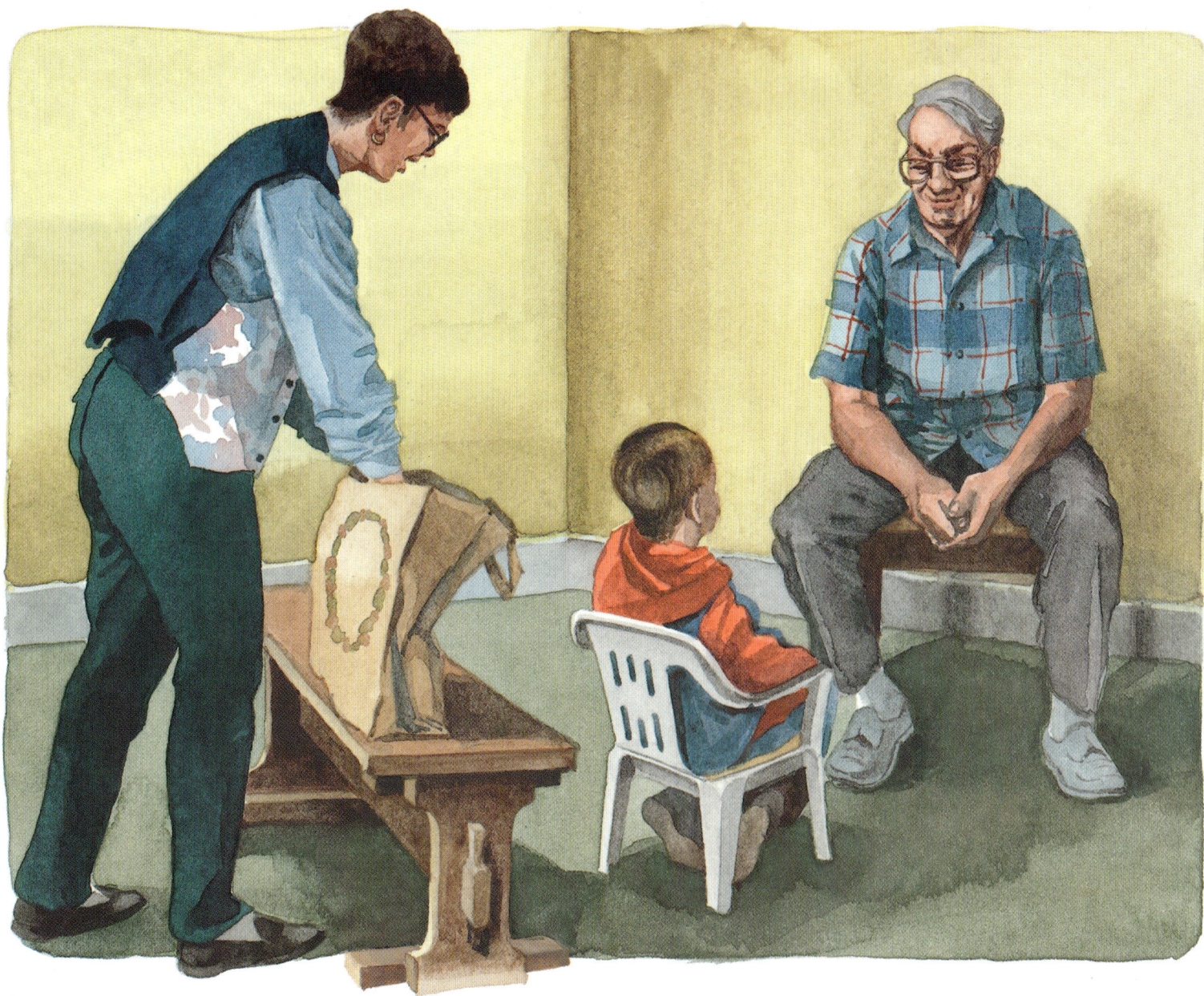

"I'm sorry that you won't have the helicopter to follow you back home, but you will see the crane," said Uncle George. "Yes," said James. "Goodbye, and thank you for having us."

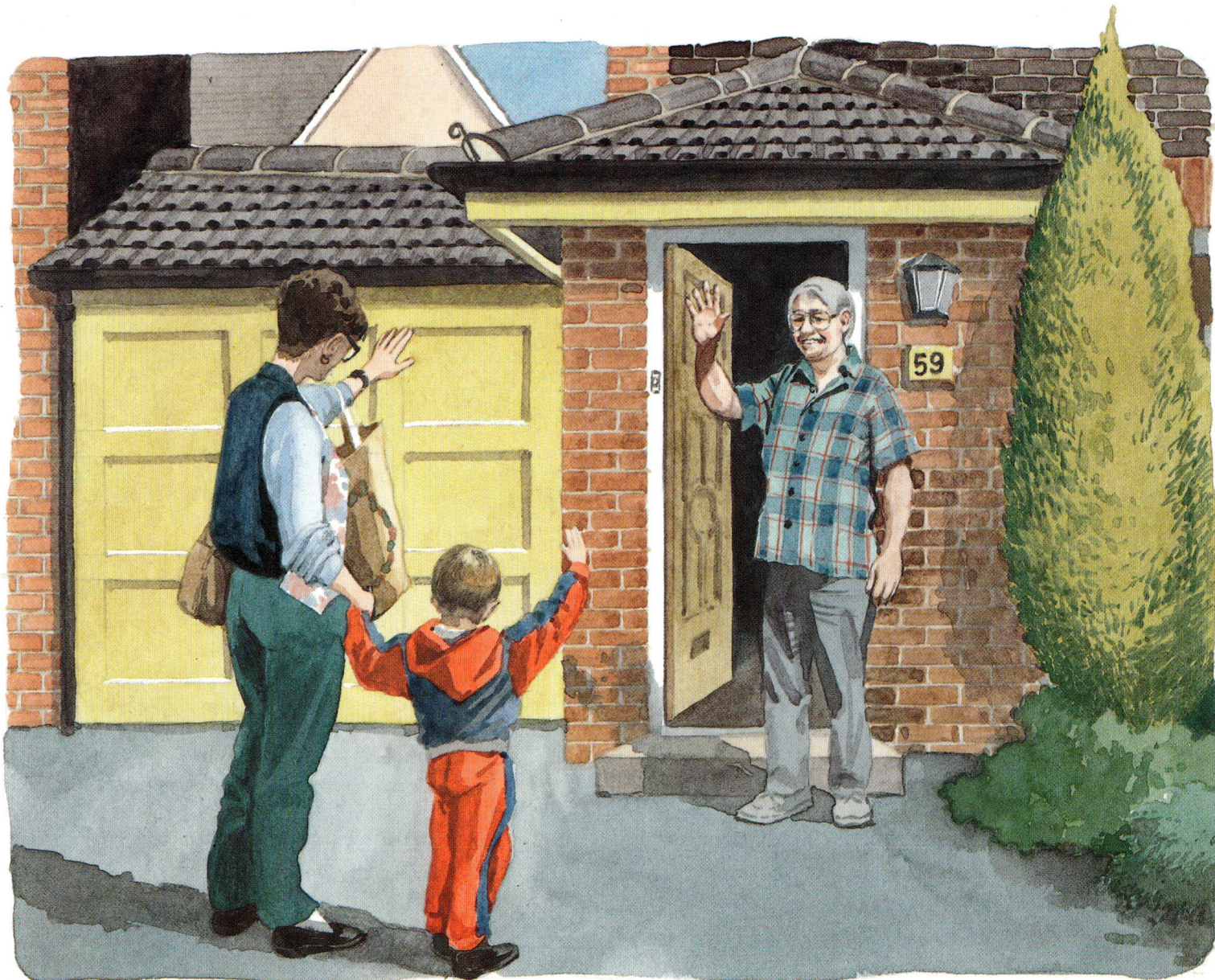

"Goodbye!" waved Uncle George, "come and see me again soon."

James soon spotted the subway and said he wanted to walk down the slope rather than use the steps, even though it meant walking a little farther to get there.

Roadwise Question

Why are you safe from traffic in a subway?

"We don't even have to look for cars when we're in the subway as there aren't any," laughed James.

"No," said his mother "we are safe in the subway. If there is a subway we should always use it so that we are safe when crossing to the other side of the road."

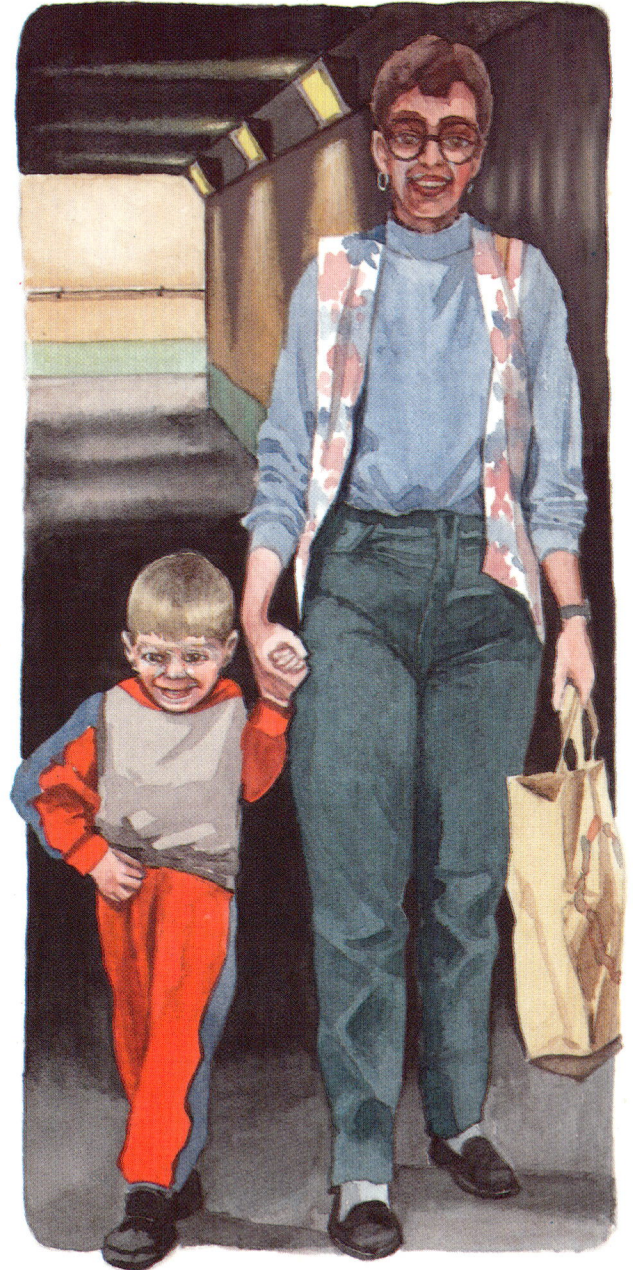

James was feeling a little tired by the time they reached the footbridge and said he would like to walk up the gentle slope, so slowly yet safely, they reached the top of the bridge.

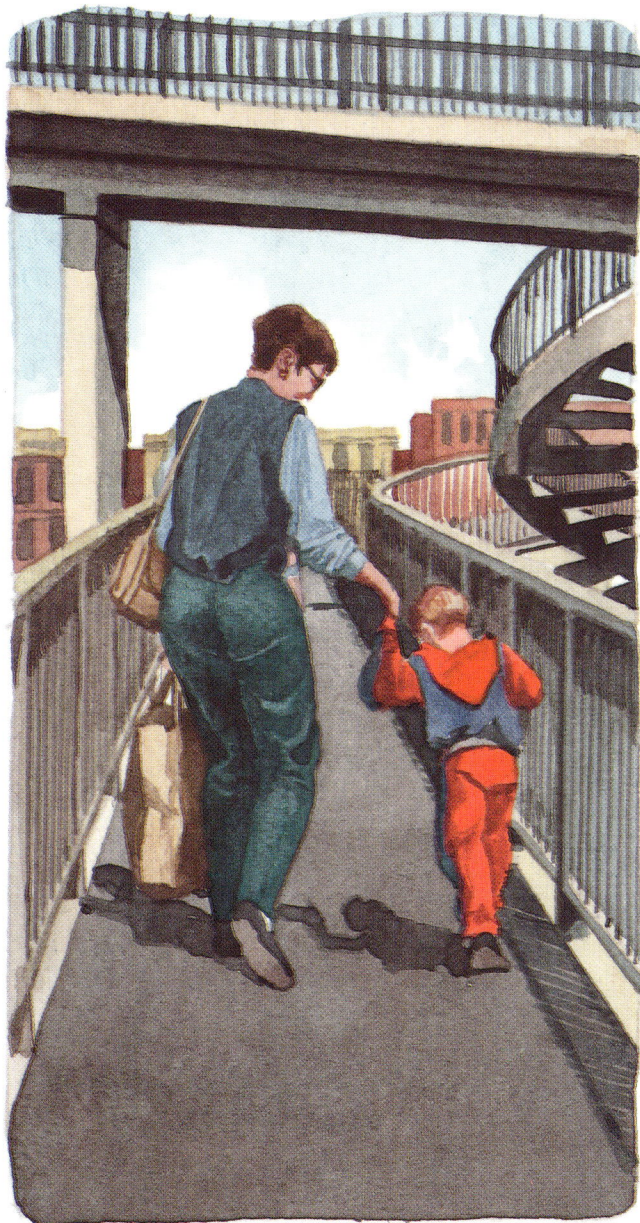

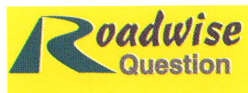

Roadwise Question Why are you safe from traffic on a footbridge?

"The crane is still working," said James as they watched it move pipes from one place to another.

James loved looking at what there was to see from the top of the bridge. "It's well worth the effort of walking up here," said James.

"Yes," said his mother "and it is a safe way to cross a road. Come on, James, we must get home."

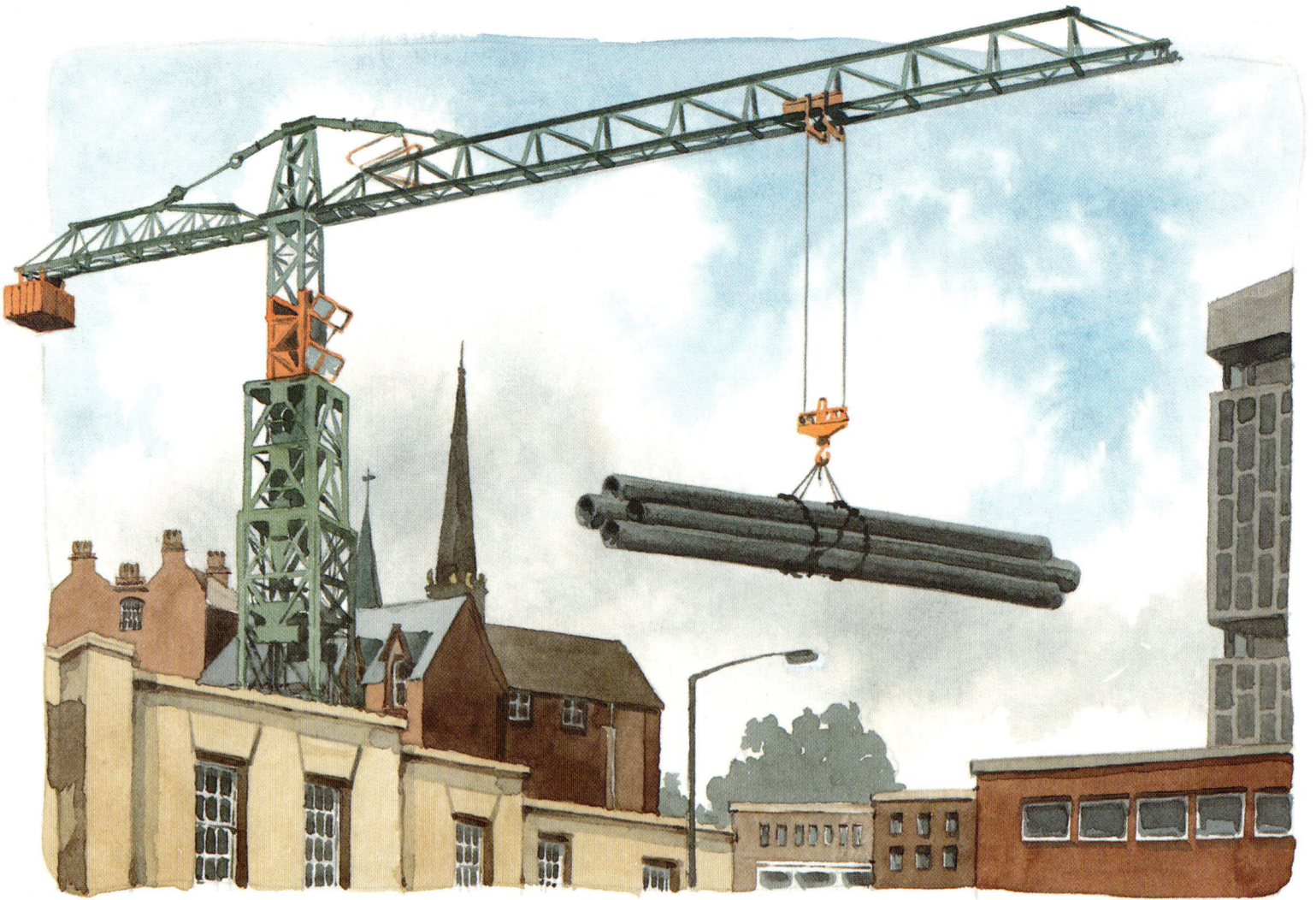

QUESTIONS RELATING TO THE USE OF FOOTBRIDGES AND SUBWAYS

These questions can be used to stimulate discussion: to help assess a child's responses the answers should be covered up.

In the story James was learning to cross a road using a footbridge and a subway. FOOTBRIDGES go from one side of a road to the other by going above the traffic. SUBWAYS take you from one side of a road to the other by going under a road with the traffic above you.

Let's look at the story again.

The first time James and his mother went up the footbridge James was feeling full of energy. Did they get to the top of the bridge by using the steps or slope?

ANSWER is on page 9.

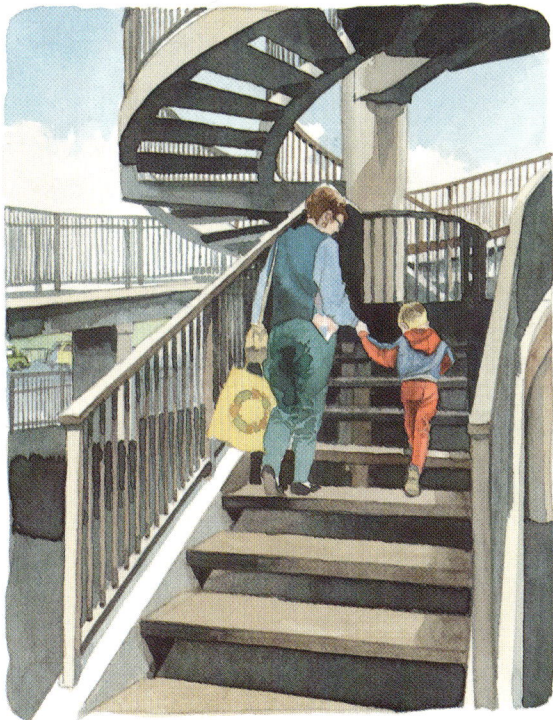

When you use a footbridge do you get to the top of the bridge by using the steps or the slope?

ANSWER Both are safe, it depends if you are tired or have lots of energy!

What appeared above James and seemed to follow them to Uncle George's home?

ANSWER is on page 12.

What have you seen from the top of a footbridge?

Look at this picture. What is there to help us cross the road?
Look and see:

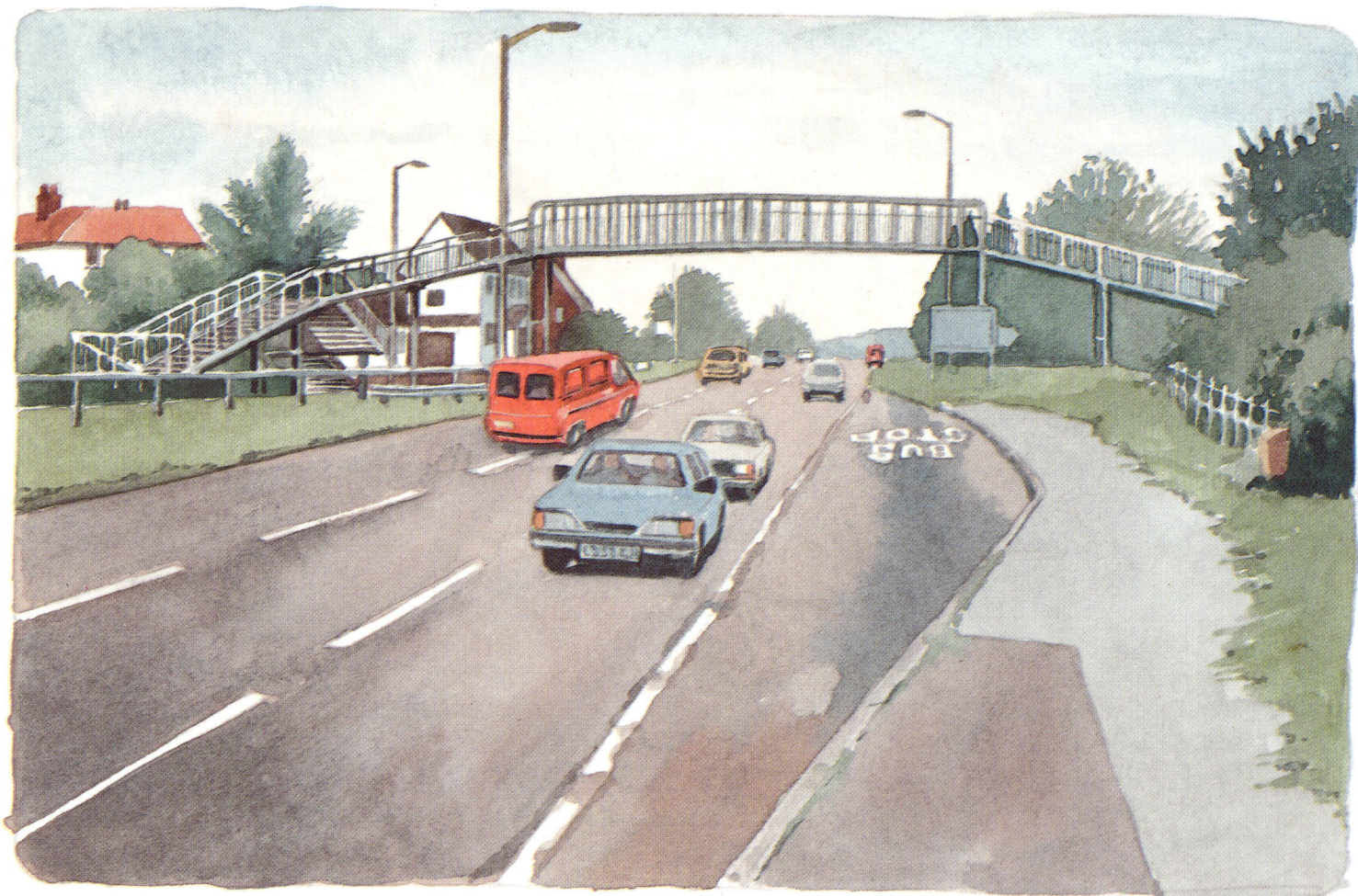

ANSWER The footbridge would be a safe place to cross the road.

When James used subways, did he prefer to go down the steps or the slope?

ANSWER James preferred the slope, see page 14.

Which do you prefer to use the steps or the slope?

Look at this picture. What is there to help us cross the road?
Look and see:

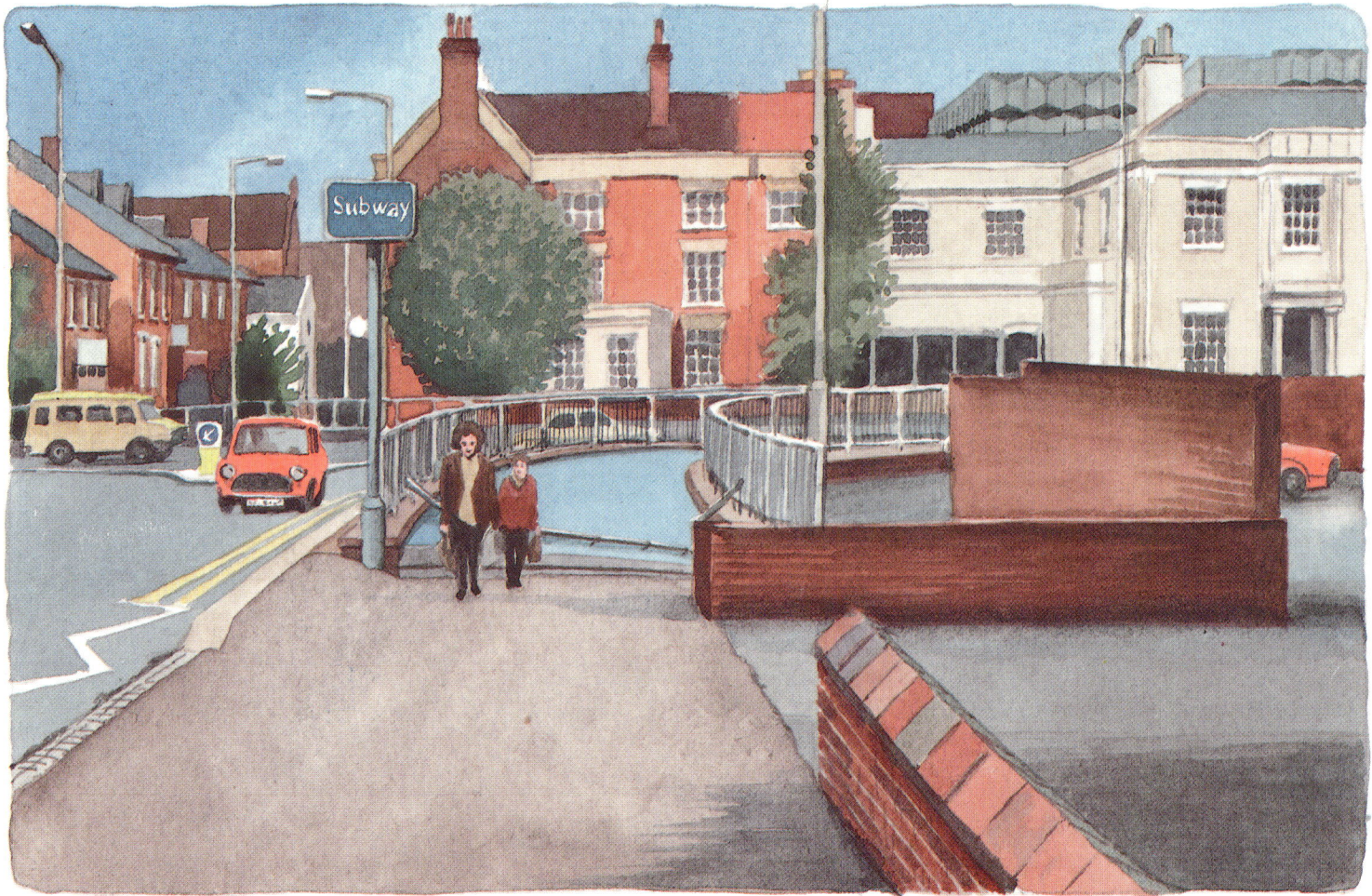

 ANSWER The subway would be a safe place to cross the road.

The Road Crossing Song

Chorus

© Words and Music by Jean Roberts
Arranged by Blodwen Roberts

Brightly

An audio cassette and the "On the Way" Music Activity Book for Teachers are available.

Verse

Spoken by reader of story, or teacher - " Is there a Footbridge or a Subway ? "
Response by child or pupils - " Yes ! "

Actions : Walking on the spot or forwards, arms swinging high

Walk a long the pave - ment and up on to the
D   **G**

Head held high, hand at forehead looking down

bridge. We can see so ma - ny things as we
D   **A**7   **D**

Walking on the spot or forwards,

safe - ly cross the road.   If we go
E7   **A**7   **D**

arms swinging low   Head held lower, body bent slightly

down be - low, the traf - fic rush - ing all a - bove.
A   **A**7   **D**   **D**7   **G**

Walking on the spot or forwards, head held high, arms swinging naturally

As we cross the road.
A   **A**7   **D**

A different verse is included in each of the four books in the "On the Way" series.

31

Acknowledgements

Many people have given helpful advice by reading draft materials,
spending time modelling for photographs, trialling materials in schools
and helping in many other ways.

My special thanks to Margaret, Biddy, Winifred, Hilary, Eleanor, José and
Arnie, Jennifer and Mitchell, David, Barbara,
Don, Yvonne, Christine, the nursery unit at Benson Junior and Infant
School and Tenterfields Primary School.